Eloquent

By

DOLLY SEN

Published by:
Chipmukapublishing
PO Box 6872
Brentwood
Essex
CM13 1ZT
United Kingdom

www.chipmunkapublishing.com

DOLLY SEN BIOG

Dolly Sen was born on 23rd October 1970 in London, where she still lives.

"I had my first psychotic experience aged 14 and stopped going to school. A series of dead end jobs followed. Pretty early on I decided I didn't want any more of the 9-5 shit and spoon race, and began to write... and maybe watch 70s cop shows."

Dolly Sen is a writer, director, artist, film-maker, poet, performer, raconteur, playwright, mental health consultant, music-maker and public speaker. Since her much-acclaimed book 'The World is Full of Laughter' was published by Chipmunka in 2002, she has had 3 further books published, had a succession of performance roles around Europe and places like The Young Vic, Trafalgar Square and The Royal Festival Hall; did a poetry tour and won a poetry award from Andrew Motion; directed two plays and several films, appeared on TV, and has done spoken word at City Hall and Oxford University.

This is staggering since she dropped out of school at 14 and has no formal qualifications. She has also had to share her life with severe mental health problems. She was told she would never amount to anything but would end up in jail or Broadmoor and she believed this and was on her way there when she changed her belief into the one of believing she could do anything she wanted to do.

This proves that the mind is an amazing thing; it can drive you mad and inspire you in the same breath. And that you can do anything if you believe you can do it.

FROM ELOQUENT CATATONIA (2001)

BALLS TO YOU

Bureaucracy is the cancer
of society's bollocks
But now the tumours are bigger
than the balls
So let us be eunuchs with
credit cards debts
and 1% of our dreams fulfilled
And say we have lived well.

EGO

I am the drowning fish
I am the bird the skies abhor
I am the rain that laughs
I am the star illuming its own darkness
I am the road leading back here again
I am the mountain feeling small
I am the ocean without a shore
I am the pain that can no longer feel itself
I am the fire too cold
I am... without you.

VALIUMSUN

Where is my Valium sun?
Which construes
eternal destitution
of my finite soul
My life, my
Irrelevant, serrated
placebo
Blowing bubbles to a
dead moon
Dark Misanthropy turns
into the sunny smiles of death
Let the Valium sun shine
on my narcoleptic lust for life.
I will look straight into it
until the whole world goes black

THE BLACK DOG

Churchill called his depression 'the black
dog'
But I love my black dog
Sometimes she is my only friend
She greets me every morning with a wag of
his tail
Like a noose seeking embrace
My barking black dog annoys
my neighbours – I like that.
My black dog can perform tricks
'Come on, girl, fetch,
fetch pain so I can throw it away
for you to bring it back again.'
I take her for long walks;
she matches me step for step
My black dog is as free as the rope around
her neck
Let sleeping dogs lie
Let sleeping dogs cry
Let sleeping dogs die.

12

LIFE'S FAIR

A heart inside a sun inside an empty
universe
Madness is an amusement park for one
Haunting, paining, strange music and lights
Ghost trains never seeing the light of day
Happy, smiling conman call:
'Try your luck in the game of life.
Loads of prizes to be won.'
But it is a rigged game; you only
get what they want to give you.
Any prize you do win is worth
less than the admission
    -   cheap, useless, but guaranteed
entertain your little soul.
But, more importantly, make
you forget you've been conned at all.

FAMILY ALBUM

Family album
Snapshots – Portraits – People
Forced smiles for posterity
The real smiles lost
somewhere in the strange, radiant
cannibalism of time, a time that
bblows sunlit bubbles through
concrete walls.
Read the freeze framed eyes
Read their blank pages of life
know that their time in waiting room
have accepted death.
The last portrait in the family album
Beautiful
Beautiful
Capturing the essence of the soul:
the last picture was a row of empty chairs.
Only death was smiling.

DEAD ON MY FEET

When I was waiting at the bus stop,
Dead on my feet,
I saw a one-legged drunk, begging
on the street, get up and put on
his false leg back-to-front.
Already unsteadied by drink, his
one leg pointing forward, and one
leg pointing backward, he didn't
know if he was coming or
going. I knew the feeling. So we
shared a bottle of wine I had,
and talked about the beginning
of the universe in the rain,
until the pubs opened and life
couldn't lie to our faces.

COFFEE MOURNING

Woke up,
& realized over coffee
my soul is dead.
How did I come to this
stunningly half-hearted
conclusion, which will not
make a dent in the world
around me: I don't remember
my dreams any more,
or even want to.
God, you learn something new
every day.

CUT

I want to feel
something –
Self-service
ECT

On the other hand,
a razor will also get
blood out of the stone
until my cup
overflows

Hell for leather;
I have torn up suicide notes for skin

See this strait-jacket,
Well—used,
abused,
almost torn at the seams,

POETRY ON THE TUBE

Madman
Tube train
Gibberish
Sitting on a bench crying for all
the one-legged pigeons of this world.
'Life fucking life!' he snarled,
before saying, 'After you,' as we both
got on the same tube
train of stale human humid silence.
'Ahhhh!' he suddenly called out.
'Jesus is an eggcup
sunflower – doodlebuf – turnip
magicman!'

He took the words
right out of my mouth.

3AM

3AM is an evil time
3AM holds my mind hostage
and nothing and no-one
can pay the ransom.
3AM every day
means the perfection
of slow madness.
3AM believes in no-one's
lies, I mean life.
3AM is on commission:
it wants my head
on a platter, to be
handed to cannibalistic
gods who have lost their appetite.
3AM is silence's dirty called
leaving obscene messages
on the answering machine of my mind.
3AM is the darkest point
before the dawn
any dawn
every dawn, a dawn
that holds a sun
slowly getting darker
3AM becomes
3:01

Salvation in impotence.

THE BIRD FEEDER

Sitting on a park bench
a carrier bag of crumbs
and a lonely man
feeding the pigeons.
This is the only way
he can express his compassion
without getting rejected.
Compassion.
Loneliness.
And birds flapping in the sunlight.

NEURONES CHEWING BONES

Why is the world full of purple Santa
Clauses
playing syphilitic pinball?
The walls are turning into clouds.
The window has become a sun
The kindest of gods make no promises.
I almost had the answer.
But the brain is a strange instrument;
it receives endless messages of pain,
But the horrible thing about it is that
it's sometimes the sender, too – not
unlike making dirty, threatening
phone calls to yourself.
And this poem is one of them.

BAD JOKE

Dedicated to death
- may he make fools of us all
just like his good friend Life.
Life makes us vicious clowns
for God to laugh at and pity.
God has a twisted sense of humour.
He makes us see life as a bad joke,
so we seek death as peace.
From transient fools in life,
we are eternal fools in death,
entertaining oblivion with its eyes closed.
The only way to fight back is
to say, 'I get the joke.' And
laugh back at the awful stand-up
comic that is existence, and when
he departs the stage
throw shit in his face.
Now *that's* funny.

ABERRATION

For madmen and maenads
the book of sanity is
a boring read. I only like to look
at the pictures. I only listen
to the celestial raconteur
of stars in its
high velocity
stillness, in its
hedonistic solitude.
Disconnect from reality.
Disconnect from the electric
chair that's saying it's keeping
the seat warm for you.
Hide from reality, because it
ultimately gets its orders
from it's boss – death.

RISE & SHINE

I woke up before the sun rose
Thoughts of suicide were my alarm
clock in those early hours.
Suicide was a comfortable bed
A sleep that actually slept
A sun that didn't burn you as it
offered your lonely world light.
Well, that morning, I wanted
death more than daytime TV. But
my gun was in another room, far
away, and as I am a lazy
person, and as my cowardice
has a beautiful star,
I waited for the sun to rise instead.

THE ANGEL

I'm in a cheap room with wallpaper older
than me,
with life and death older than me.
This cheap room with more worth than me.
Insomnia
loves to decorate interiors, it likes to
paint horror and death in beautiful colours.
Munch's work are mere cartoon characters
compared.
Insomnia's gargoyles smile at me, making
lewd comments I've heard a million times
before,
and my mind is thinking happy, happy shiny
thoughts
of the blackest of deaths.
Anyway, out of nowhere, an angel appeared
in my room.
First I thought: great another weirdo,
another
burglar coming to steal what I no longer
own.
When I saw its golden wings outspread,
then I
thought: what bad taste to bring purity
into a sullen habitat, like a newborn baby
into this beautiful world. But I must admit
it was better than seeing a pink elephant
take a shit in my room.

The angel looked down at me, 'It's time,' he said.

'Time for what?'

'Shit, you're alive!'

'unfortunately, yes.'

'I must have got the wrong address. I was looking for
a 75 year old senile incontinent with
a mustache and bad breath.'

'Oh, Mrs Glover, she lives next door.'

'Sorry about this,' he apologized, 'I'd better go.'

'No, don't go – take me instead. Her next door can wait.'

'No, I am here for Mrs Glover.'

'No, take me, life is too painful.'

'Yeah, for you and six billion others.
Besides, God's waiting for her next door,
and I think you are wanted at the other place.'

'I am already at the other place. Anyway, why Mrs Glover?'

She's a bitch, she throws shit and piss at my window.'

'Yeah,' the angel chuckled, 'but her heart's in the right place.'

'Ok, piss off then.'

'Once again, sorry for waking you.
Remember, God
loves you.'

'Yeah, right,' I say, unconvinced.

So the angel went next door
and left me alone
to stare at the lonely, empty walls again.

DEATHBED INSOMNIA

Dying
Slowing down
My father's body
felt no pain
As it approached its own
bored demise
   -   just useful lethargy that'll
melt into the sun to dream
dreams not hindered nor
invalidated by the catatonic
dynamics of the breathing soul.
He looks into our eyes
and says
'You will never grow old,'
Is this some strange,
pained,
magical,
apologetic statement of the dying?

No, it's an ordinary fact
his eyes will remember
When it gazes into its permanent
purple amnesia. We say
goodbye, but he does not
see us leave. He has gone.
His face – the mask of a chaotic
puppet – is still looking for something.
Time has passed for us, but not for
him. Time just withered the only set

of flowers on his grave.
Somehow he belongs there:
Life did not suit him; he didn't know
what to do with it, except make us
wish he was where he is now.

NOW TIME FOR A COMMERCIAL BREAK

Now a word from our sponsors – Samsara
Buy now, pay eternity
One seat in heaven
Available in blue

Your soul must go,
With a new and improved
Recipe for death.

Karma – a great bargain
Buy one life, get one free.

CALLING TIME

Lone woman
in a bar full of men
They leave her alone
    -   no pick-ups
or drunken flirting.
Any idea of that died
when they saw her eyes,
The horrible myopic stare
through loneliness cataracts of pain
'Smile,' some useless human
being being useless said to her.
She did try, but half a weak
smile made her pain uglier
and her face
even harder to look at.

This bar has no karaoke.
No satellite TV.
No conversation.
It's not that kind of bar.
What the hell could you say
to death over a drink?
Gazes do not touch each other
No one looks each other
in the eye,
Including their own
Especially their own

The soul
Minus its dreams
Minus its hope
Minus itself
Comes here to drink.

REVERIE

I've lost my ability to dream
The bloody things give me headache,
anyway.
They feed the obscene hunger of hope
- and he is a fat bastard now anyway
     who
can't even be bothered to get out of bed.
My dreams lack total imagination
Nothing happens
I won't allow it to
Far too fucking painful
Cowardice has to wake up to a new day,
you see.

AVERAGE HUMAN BEING

I'm a sadist who doesn't want to hurt
anyone.
I'm a killer who believes all life is precious.
I'm an obsessive-compulsive who is a lazy
old cow,
I'm a loving person full of hate,
A shiteater full of good taste
A sinner with a puritanical streak
I'm nobody's slave but I cannot do what I
want
I'm special in my anonymity,
another face in a faceless world.
I'm just your average human being.

THE HOLY ATHEIST

I have a friend, Joe. I call
Joe the holy atheist. He hated
that but his heart is bigger
than the smallest star.
There was this one guy, an
ex-psychiatric patient, driven
by God know what ghosts, would
spend the whole day walking,
pushing on and on. I think
he was trying to escape humanity.
He would reject any money or food
offered to him. Joe, the holy atheist,
saw the man's soul, I mean sole was
wearing thin. Guessing the size, he
bought a 2nd pair of shoes. When Joe
saw the man again, he stopped him.
All the man saw was another human being.
'Oh, no, pain, more pain.' He thought.
Joe sat him down, changed his shoes
and smiled.
The man smiled back.
Life is hell
But you do get the occasional smile.

His heart would break whenever he saw
a one-legged pigeon or a stray skinny dog.
He went to nursing homes, where
stroke-ridden souls would sit unable to
talk, move or even cry; hugging only

caused them physical pain.
Joe would take their grubby spectacles and
wipe them clean.
Nature is the ultimate truth,
but occasionally it tells lies.

On one of his park bench meditations,
he'd tell me we were all soiled gods, that
before our births we were celestial beings,
who wanted bodies to swap divinity for a
dick
Moksha for money. Planet earth was
ex-gods anonymous, he said.
No, he added, no God is worth one dying
Child's scream.
In a godless world occasionally there is
divinity.

One night a man was beating on his
girlfriend. Joe stepped in.
'Fuck off!' the man said.
'Yeah, fuck off!' the woman added.
But he wouldn't. There would be no pain.
Joe was being unreasonable, because
the man stabbed Joe in the heart.
How could he miss, it was such a
big target.
He didn't make it.
Eternal life is beautiful, but occasionally
you have to watch it die.

FLIGHT

My mind is in flight
So high it's looking down at birds
It's looking down at clouds
It's even looking down on earth
People have totally disappeared from view
You realize how small they really are
I am flying higher and higher
Thoughts have turned the speed of light
a loser to a snail, to a rain running
backwards
I am so high, this solar system is a service
station
on the road to newer stars
I am so high,
when I come back down to earth
it will be a dead empty thing, a million
miles into the future
So I think I will stay where I am.

SHIT AND CHOCOLATE ICE CREAM

The trouble is
people don't know
the difference between shit
and chocolate ice cream

More bills in the post
I just want to be treated like a human
being.
Then I realize they *are* treating
me like a human being.
It's days like these
which makes a gun in the mouth
taste like a fucking lollipop.

Life is shit, but it's a good job
shit looks like chocolate ice
cream, I told a friend.

The glass is half-empty for
you, my friend replied, it's
half full for me.
half-empty or half-full,
what's the fucking difference,
it's still piss in the glass.

DEATH DISCO

Death disco
Dance on your own grave
plagiarise a billion deaths:
Close your eyes and see
your dreams disappoint you
See your cowardice pampered
into mental obesity
where other people
point and stare
unawares
that they're walking though a
universe that is nothing
but a desiccated mirror
divested of the light
we perpetually keep
in
the
dark

DEAD SOULS

The poetry of demons
speaks
in uneasy sleep
too easily.
It gives my mind
futile genius
A genius that'll make
a bloody mess
of someone's carpet
some day.
I am God inside the body
of a nobody
But then again, aren't we all?

These voices in my head
get my undivided attention.
They dictate my suicide note
to me on the most beautiful of days,

Poetic justice.

They tear my mind apart;
they rent out my mind
to dead souls,
dead souls that were happy
to be dead.
But when I hear nothing
but silence,
I miss them.

Insane, isn't it?

OUR DAZE

Even encased
In that bloody-thirsty tomb,
I walked on eggshells,
sunrises bleeding
underfoot.
The yoke seeped and ran,
embryo logically
convulsed
draining blood
from my heart made
of home – demolished
to accommodate
further wasteland suns
that milk and leech
and scorch a mirage
egotism,
that bleeds the ghost
inside of me.

HEART

I seek the percussive intangibility,
impossibility of your heart.
My heart, on the other hand, is a pool
of gasoline. Light a match, come on,
take a closer look.
Every sunrise immolates itself,
engendering this genocide of one
Leaving me with
Adrenalised
Sexualized
Alienation
Leaving crying with teargas joy
Leaving me with the paraphernalia
of contorted flowers
Or maybe you are only leaving me...

CAGE

I want my mind to have wings
& fly away from here, leave
my body behind, I don't mind.
I don't want my
Thoughts to be calcine birds
In every sunrise
Life stole my wings; death
hasn't promised to return them.
So if my mind has wings, it will
be a deaf, dumb and blind bird
begging for a cage to be safe in.
This cage of skin
This cage of bone
This cage of eyes
This cage of stone alone.

THE JOYS OF CHILDHOOD

The joys of childhood
were outside my window
Not where I lived.
Looking out of the window
to where other children played
became too painful; I preferred TV
or dreaming of death.

Games at school: last one picked
boy, did I feel the preciousness of life
there, of playing games designed to make
Me
Odd
One
Out.
I was never really any good
at games; nobody
ever asked me to play.
I was never really any good at
being a child; nobody ever
asked me to be one.

WAITING

I do not fear death
But I do not like to leave you
behind in life – alone.
I can say my last breath
will join the winds – that sounds nice.
When it touches your skin, it's
saying, 'Feel, feel life.'
My eyes will be flowers
in your garden
watching over you. My touch
will join the ocean & wash away
your pain. I lied
when I said I don't fear
death; I am scared to death
of death, of anything
that will take me
away from you.
I'll be here and you'll
be there, in another
world. But death
is nothing but a waiting room.
God is no one but the old man
in the corner without
a thing to say.

But that's where I'll be
Waiting
Waiting

Don't take too long...

www.ingramcontent.com/pod-product-compliance
Lightning Source LLC
Chambersburg PA
CBHW031934080426
42734CB00007B/678